An Easy Way
To Understand
Detoxing
For Men And Women

Also By Brian B Jacques

His very popular Series of Mini-Health Books includes:

- An Easy Way To Understand Eczema and Psoriasis
- An Easy Way To Understand Stress and Depression
- An Easy Way To Understand Vitamins and Minerals
- An Easy Way To Understand Parasites, Worms, Candida, Constipation & Detoxing
- An Easy Way To Understand Crohn's Disease and IBD
- An Easy Way To Understand Body Building For Men And Women
- An Easy Way To Understand Alzheimer's Disease
- An Easy Way To Understand Herpes
- An Easy Way To Understand Parkinson's Disease
- An Easy Way To Understand Autism In Children
- An Easy Way To Understand Fibromyalgia
- An Easy Way To Understand Your Body Systems
- An Easy Way To Understand Erectile Dysfunction
- An Easy Way To Understand Heart Disease, High Blood Pressure & Stroke
- An Easy Way To Understand Detoxing For Men & Women
- How To Lose Weight After 40
- How To Lose Weight And Maintain Your Ideal Weight Permanently
- Amino Acids & Enzymes—What Are They & Why Do You Need Them
- The Little A–Z Dictionary of Herbal Remedies
- The Magic Of Vitamins & Minerals
- Effective Methods To Stop Smoking
- Eat Wholefoods And Take Supplements—The Ultimate Lifestyle Guide
- Stress Busters Adult Coloring Book

All these books are available as Kindle Editions (available from the Kindle Store on Amazon.com, and other countries Amazon sites where the Kindle platform is supported.) Many of these books are also available for the Barnes and Noble "Nook". In addition, many of these titles are available as print editions from the Amazon website.

An Easy Way
To Understand
Detoxing
For Men And Women

Brian B Jacques

Wisdom For Life Media

Publisher: Wisdom For Life Media (www.wisdomforlifemedia.com)

While they have made every effort to verify the information provid-ed in this publication, neither the author nor the publisher assumes any responsibility for errors in, omissions from, or different inter-pretation of the subject matter.

The information herein may be subject to varying laws, regulations, and practices in different areas, states and countries. The purchaser or reader assumes all responsibility for use of the information.

All information included within this book is for educational pur-poses only. The author and publishers do not attempt to diagnose or treat any medical conditions, be it to do with health, diet or exercise.

If you consider that you have any kind of medical condition, then, you should consult a qualified medical practitioner or doctor or qualified naturopathic doctor before starting any herbal, vitamin and/or mineral program or supplement regime, exercise or health training program or diet suggested in this book.

This book is not intended for anyone under the age of 18 years, nor is it intended for breast feeding or pregnant women, underweight people or anyone with eating disorders or a health condition that requires special diets or medical treatment.

The author and publishers disclaim any liability for any loss however caused by anyone using the information contained in this book.

Images are either copyright the author or are used under the terms of a Royalty Free Agreement.

ISBN - 13: 978-1547031337

ISBN - 10: 1547031336

Published in The United States of America.

"Education is the kindling of a flame, not the filling of a vessel." —Socrates

Contents

Acknowledgment

To the many people I have come into contact with throughout my life, whose belief in me has made everything possible and worthwhile.

Introduction

So what are toxins, and where do they come from? Toxins take two forms (external and internal) and impact various parts of the body.

The external part comprises what we breathe in and what we eat and drink—usually a Western diet which is high in fats, sugars and chemicals and low in fiber. Other factors include: a lack of exercise, constipation, use of various medications as well as other lifestyle choices.

The internal part comprises the metabolic by-products of the diet. When the body digests food it creates toxic wastes. When the body is in healing and repairing mode it creates toxic wastes. If you experience negative emotions like anger and stress the body will create toxins.

These poisons build up in the colon, liver, kidneys and blood, in addition to causing inflammation in joint tissue which can lead to arthritis. Usually the early visible sign of toxins is when an eruption occurs on the surface of the skin. This can be in the form of pimples, blackheads, puss spots and other skin conditions.

Longer term, major health issues could arise such as chronic fatigue, depression, diabetes, heart, kidney and liver disease or cancer. Premature aging could also be a concern.

All these toxic factors impact the immune system which is the body's protection mechanism against disease. When the immune system is not working properly, it is then unable to protect the body against airborne invaders which enter through the nose, mouth and skin as well as metabolic changes within the body's structure.

Parasites and worms are often present when there is a toxic build-up in the body. These "invaders" are not your friends, and are only too happy to reside—usually in your colon, when a toxic environment is present. I have covered this subject in some detail, and have described various drug treatments that may be prescribed by your physician, as well as more natural alternative in the form of herbal remedies, which have been used for centuries to treat this problem.

In this book I have covered various detox programs for your consideration—several of these have their own celebrity followers. Some of these involve using various fruits and vegetables which you probably already have in your kitchen, others—such as herbal detoxing involves purchasing herbal products either from a health food store or on the Internet.

Whichever detoxing program you decide to use, before commencing, it is important to discuss this with your physician to make sure what you propose doing is right for you. This is especially important if you are pregnant or breast feeding, or if you have any prior medical conditions and/or are taking any type of medication. It is important to ensure that any herbal remedies you propose taking do not conflict with any of your medications.

1. Good Colon Health

Consuming the typical Western diet means that many Americans suffer from poor colon health, and unfortunately many are not aware of it. The condition of the stool that is excreted gives a good indication of the health of the colon. A good stool pattern requires the ability to eliminate two or three stools that are formed each day. The first stool which should also be the longest should be expelled in the morning; a stool half of this size should be expelled later the same day. When eliminating stools there should be no straining involved; the stool should be expelled without any effort.

Constipation causes a build-up of stool in the colon wall, which does not bode well for good health. This build-up of fecal matter which may have been there for many years, can cause inflammation in the colon, with the result that a decaying effect is triggered, which causes a toxic build-up causing other tissues and organs of the body to be affected, as it travels throughout the bloodstream. This condition can cause the intestinal wall to leech bacteria and viruses into the bloodstream, which can result in various chronic illnesses in the body.

In fact the colon is one of the major areas in the body where toxins reside, and if it is left untreated, then, it becomes a breeding ground for all kinds of unfriendly bacteria, parasites, worms and amoeba like structures all of which have one purpose—to do your body harm. They are not your friends.

Many people who undertake a colon cleanse often lose as much as 7–9 pounds in body weight. This is all impacted toxic matter that has been purged out of the system, along with any parasites that reside there.

It is not difficult to maintain good colon health. One of the most effective things you can do is to increase your fiber intake, as well as eating more fruits and vegetables. Fiber is one of the best ways to help prevent constipation. The ideal daily dietary fiber intake should be 38 grams for men and 25 grams for women.

This figure is based on adults less than 50 years of age. If you are over 50 then men should consume 30 grams of fiber each day and women 21 grams. It is also important to consume at least eight glasses of filtered water each day to help the fiber work more effectively, and in addition, it also helps prevent a hard stool which can result in constipation.

In addition, doing a regular exercise program at least 3 to 4 times a week for 30 minutes each time will also help to stimulate all your body systems, which can also have a positive effect on colon health.

Laxatives should be used sparingly and not as a regular daily occurrence. Additionally, do not ignore your body's urge to have a bowel movement. If you do, this can cause a lazy colon which can lead to constipation.

If you think you are constipated then you could try drinking prune juice or eating prunes before deciding on laxatives. And also remember to add fiber and water to your diet.

If you have persistent constipation it is probably a good idea to consult your physician to determine there are no other underlying health issues which may be causing the problem.

2. How To Do A Detox

Human beings are mobile depositories for literally hundreds of different chemicals and toxins that in this modern age have become part of our homes and offices, so says the Environmental Protection Agency (EPA), whose statements have been backed up by the majority of naturopathic physicians.

According to the EPA the air in our homes is more toxic than the air outside—even than in inner cities. This is mainly due to the fact that homes have become more airtight to improve the efficiency of air conditioning and heating systems; and that is not all, we are also bringing more cleaning chemicals into our homes as well.

Detoxing can take various forms from a simple colon cleanse to fasting and making significant changes to lifestyle choices. The body is a remarkable living thing, in that it has the ability to heal itself when given adequate nutrients and the tools it needs to do the job.

Sadly, the average Western diet is lacking in these nutrients and many synthetically manufactured vitamin and mineral supplements aren't always as bioavailable to the body as they should be. Bioavailable means that the supplements should be available to the body in much the same way that nutrients from food are.

A detoxification program basically means cleansing the body of toxins and chemicals that prevents it from maintaining optimum health. By expelling impurities—or helping the body to clear these impurities from the blood, liver, kidneys and intestines, every cell of the body will be improved. A detox program will enable the organs of the body to rest during a fastening process, thus stimulating the liver, promoting elimination, improving circulation and providing optimum fuel to the body through the addition of healthy nutrients.

The initial step in a detox process is to lighten the load on your body. During the detox, it is important to eliminate alcohol, coffee, cigarettes and refined sugars as well as saturated fats. All of these things are toxic to the body and provide obstacles in the healing process. It is also important to either eliminate or minimize the use of chemical based cleaners in the home in addition to personal care products which are ingested into the body through the skin and mucous membranes.

Additionally, it's important to look at other products in the home that are derived from plastic sources. An example of this is plastic containers made from polyvinyl chloride which releases toxic chemicals into the atmosphere. Another example is lead, although this is not so widely used today. However, in past decades lead in gasoline contributed to high levels of lead in the bones of women over the age of 40. To counteract any lead particles that may migrate into the bloodstream women should ensure they get adequate amounts of calcium, magnesium, and vitamin D, as well as a implementing a regular exercise program which will help to decrease the incidence of osteoporosis, also known as brittle bone disease.

It is also a good idea to dispense with the use of air fresheners in the home. While they may give off a nice scent, they are in fact filled with neurotoxins that have the effect of coating the inside of the nose which makes it difficult for you to "smell"—in reality, they don't really eliminate odors. It is far preferable to use natural alternatives such as: opening windows, placing some beautiful plants in the home or office, and make sure you empty the garbage cans frequently.

Drinking a minimum of 4 pints of filtered water each day will help to stimulate the kidneys, liver and digestive system to work more effectively. This will also help to boost your metabolism and accelerate the elimination of toxins from the body. Including other foods such as brown rice, herbal teas, garlic, lemons, cabbage and onions in your diet will also assist your body to eliminate built-up toxins.

It is also important to add more fiber to your diet. Statistics show that the average American diet is badly lacking in adequate fiber; this has the effect of increasing toxic build-up in the cells as well as an increased incidence of constipation. Also organically grown fruits and vegetables will assist in elimination and cleansing of the colon. In addition, you can help to improve the function of the liver by using various herbs such Milk Thistle and Dandelion Root as well as drinking green tea. Increasing your levels of vitamins C. will assist the body in producing glutathione—an antioxidant which is another compound that helps to eliminate toxins and prevent premature aging, in addition to warding off chronic disease.

Stress is often a major factor in everyday life, but it is also another toxin to the body. Stress has a negative impact on the liver and kidneys, as well as the circulatory system; it can cause increased hypertension (high blood pressure). All of these problems can be precursors to more serious health issues. By reducing the stress in your life and promoting more positive emotional feelings you will go a long way in helping to detoxifying your lifestyle.

You may consider beginning your toxic detoxifying process by going on a fast. Nutritionists believe that fasting for 24 hours every two weeks or one month is actually very healthy for the body. In modern times we actually very rarely go hungry, but in past centuries when we had to forage for all our food, days may go by with nothing to eat at all. This in effect was a natural fasting process, and we can replicate this today by doing a modern-day fast involving drinking filtered water and juices made from organic fruits and vegetables. Doing this, you'll rest your liver and intestines enabling them to work more efficiently.

Did you know that sweat and perspiration is used by the body as a means of eliminating toxins? You can assist the body's toxin elimination process with the use of saunas, exercise and hot showers which all have the effect of eliminating waste material from the body. Dry brushing your skin can also assist in removing toxins through the pores. In fact, special brushes are available for this purpose from various natural product stores.

Removing excess chemicals and toxins from the body will have a very positive impact on your overall health and well-being.

3. Consider A Cleansing Diet

A cleansing diet is an excellent way to purge your body of toxins or undigested food items. There are various cleansing diets available each with their own approach to detoxification.

Some cleansing diets are based on only eating one of two different types of foods. Some are based on only drinking liquids but no solid foods at all, while still allowing a person to eat several types of food. Then there are cleansing programs which feature various herbal combinations. So you can see there is a wide choice available so it is important for each individual to choose a cleansing diet program that they will feel comfortable with.

Every person is exposed to chemical toxins as they go about their daily life. Toxins take many forms: some are residual products of the foods that have been eaten, whilst others are classed as environmental toxins which are airborne and are breathed in. As toxins are invisible, they are often little thought about, but it is important to purge them from the body. It is a good idea to do a cleansing program at least twice a year which will help the body systems function more effectively.

As mentioned above, one type of cleansing diet involves only drinking bottled water and freshly squeezed juices. In reality, you may not wish to continue with a cleansing diet for a long period of time due to its intensity. An adequate amount of time is usually between 3 to 7 days. Of note, this type of cleanse is sometimes used prior to your physician performing tests on your lower and upper gastrointestinal tract.

Some individuals use a vegan type diet as a cleansing program. This involves eating natural fruits and vegetables. All forms of meat and carbohydrates are eliminated on this type of diet. Drinks consist of either water or freshly squeezed juices.

While on a cleansing diet if you start to feel unwell then you should start to eat something a little more substantial. It is not necessary to eat a full course meal, but only to eat something that is a bit more filling. It is also important, and indeed advisable to take a multivitamin supplement every day to make up for vitamin and mineral shortfalls in the diet whilst you're on a cleansing diet program. In addition, it is also important to drink plenty of filtered or bottled still water, and also get adequate amounts of rest and sleep.

In years gone by people rarely ate three large meals each day, as is often normal practice today. For example, farmers often ate a large breakfast and dinner but skipped lunch because they were busy in the fields all day. In addition, because of their physical activity they burnt a lot of the calories off each day. As another example, native tribes whose life revolved around hunting and gathering would frequently go for several days without food when it couldn't be found. This type of eating plan allowed the body to cleanse itself naturally.

When you are near the end of your cleansing diet program you should start to gradually introduce a variety of foods back into your body in small amount at a time. It is not a good idea to introduce everything back all at once as this could put your body into shock mode. Remember, your body has been deprived of its natural food intake for several days so it will need some time to readjust back to normal again. Eating small meals is advisable as your body readjusts back to normal. The last thing your body needs is to be weighed down with a heavy caloric intake again.

To have your body free of toxins is a worthwhile goal to aim for. A body that is loaded with toxins cannot work effectively, and it can be exposed to various ailments and health conditions if it is left in this state over time.

4. Doing A Colon Cleanse

The purpose of colon cleansing is to help reduce bloating, constipation and fatigue. There are two schools of thought regarding this subject. Those in favor believe that colon cleansing has significant health benefits, whilst many doctors on the other hand take a different view. Doctors often recommend a colon cleanse in preparation for a medical examination or surgery, but don't recommend it on a regular basis.

One of the purposes of the colon is to absorb water and sodium to help maintain the body's electrolyte balance; the danger is that regular colon cleansing can disrupt this balance, with the result that salt depletion can occur as well as dehydration. If done over a long period of time, this can lead to heart failure, anemia and malnutrition.

Many healthcare professionals recommend colon cleansing as the result of the majority of people eating a standard Western diet which is common in the US as well as many parts of Europe. This diet is high in saturated fat, meat, polyunsaturated fats and processed foods.

The problem with this type of diet is that it exposes the colon and intestines to decomposing foods for a longer period of time. This rotting food exposes an individual to a greater risk of developing intestinal diseases. Those people who enjoy a vegetarian diet have a reduced risk for developing an intestinal illness since the food they eat moves through the intestines much more quickly because animal fats are not included in the diet.

There are two main kinds of colon cleansing. The first comprises a powder or liquid supplements which works from the top down. The second is colonic irrigation or hydrotherapy which involves an enema to flush out the lower intestines with water. Holistic practitioners believe that if the colon is not kept clean, fecal waste material will build up, which will then harden and decrease the absorption of nutrients into the body. Also, these unwanted toxins and chemicals may have a negative impact on the integrity of the intestinal wall.

As these toxins and chemicals build up in the intestines, there is a danger that a build-up of bad bacteria or viruses can occur, which may cause a leaking of these viruses or bacteria into the abdominal cavity or bloodstream. Add all this together, and we have a scenario where we could have a seriously compromised intestinal system.

Using a colon cleansing program may not just involve the colon but the entire intestinal tract. This approach may assist the body to work more efficiently, and at the same time give you more energy in addition to ridding the system of all the toxins, chemicals, bad bacteria and viruses.

As mentioned in the chapter on Good Colon Health, one of the most effective colon cleanses involves including a high fiber diet possibly using psyllium husks that is low in fat and high in vitamin D. Incorporating a regular exercise program is also beneficial as it helps to move waste materials through the colon, ready for elimination.

A high fiber diet also reduces the risk of constipation. However, it is always important to remember that high fiber diets also need adequate amounts of filtered water—ideally, eight glasses per day. This will help to keep your body hydrated, as well as helping the fiber work more effectively.

To detoxify your body using colon cleanses is a personal decision for you to make. Detoxing however, is only part of the story. You also need to possibly make other lifestyle changes as well. These could include incorporating an exercise program as well as making choices in the type of foods you eat. And never forget the all-important daily liquid—ideally filtered water— your body needs to keep hydrated as well. All of these things assist your body in performing its billions of daily functions to help you enjoy your lifestyle and keep you healthy.

5. Detoxing With A Herbal Colon Cleanse

Herbal remedies have been used for centuries—long before drugs came on the scene—to treat major elements of the body. This is therefore no surprise to learn that herbs are also very effective as part of a body detoxification program.

Herbs are one of the best natural ways to undertake a colon cleanse. I have included a list at the end of this section. But briefly, herbs such as licorice root, milk thistle, horsetail, violet leaf and passionflower root as well as a fiber source such as psyllium are often used.

When undertaking a detoxing program it is important to drink plenty of filtered water to assist the liver in eliminating toxins from your body. Notice I mentioned filtered water, or if this is not possible then the best quality water you can find.

Do not use tap water. This is full of chemicals and is not good for you. It will not be very beneficial in a detoxing program. Chlorine and fluoride are often added to tap water in many states or districts and countries.

Fluoride is a by-product of aluminium processing and is highly toxic and poisonous. The aluminium industry had to dispose of this waste somehow, so they did a good "selling job" by convincing everyone that this poisonous and toxic substance was good for dental health amongst other things.

The trouble is this toxic substance ends up in the liver, kidneys and other organs where it resides in a toxic form, until it is removed with a detoxing program.

Everyone reacts to a detox in different ways. You could experience symptoms such as headaches, a sore throat, muscle aches, constipation or flu-like symptoms. These conditions are only temporary and this is the body's way of telling you that the program is working and that internal adjustments are being made.

Following on from your detox program, you should consider making some dietary adjustments, by only eating organic produce: meat, poultry, vegetables and fruits, as well as oily fish (mackerel, tuna, salmon); fish should preferably be grilled or poached, not fried.

Increase your fiber intake. Remember fiber is one of the best forms of absorbing toxins. Psyllium in particular acts like a sponge in absorbing toxins and eliminating them along with fecal matter.

Don't forget whole grains, nuts and seeds which are a good source of fiber and contain beneficial oils in addition to vitamins and minerals.

Getting adequate sleep and rest—which allows the body to repair and rejuvenate itself - as well as introducing an exercise program if you don't have one already will be beneficial to all your body systems, but especially the circulatory system.

6. Products For Herbal Detoxing

This is rather a long list. You may be well informed and able to make your own selection. If you are unsure, then you may wish to discuss this list with a naturopathic doctor or other qualified natural health care provider.

Diuretic and Laxative Herbs
Alfalfa

Alfalfa is a grass which contains all the essential amino acids as well as being rich in trace minerals and enzymes. It is frequently taken to lessen the effects of hay fever allergies. It is also fed to horses as a counter to arthritic conditions and digestive problems.

As it is a good source of fiber, it is useful for detoxifying the body in addition to improving liver health.

Cascara Sagrada

Well known for it quick acting laxative effects. It is often used for constipation in addition to helping purge toxins from the body. It promotes peristaltic action—the movement of waste matter through the colon, and stimulates secretions from the gall bladder, liver, pancreas and stomach.

Guar Gum

Is often used in fiber blends as it provides soluble digestible fiber. The body needs non-soluble as well as soluble fiber. Guar gum soaks toxins up like a sponge, has a laxative effect, curbs appetite and is beneficial in lowering cholesterol.

Hibiscus Flowers

Hibiscus flowers have anti-bacterial properties as well as being an anti-parasitic. In addition they act as a diuretic and are soothing.

Licorice Root

Licorice root provides nutritional support to the adrenal glands which is especially important when the body is under stress.

It boosts energy in addition to supporting the digestive system. It is usually added to Chinese formulas in order to bring balance and harmony to the ingredients.

In a detoxing program it will rid the body of over 1,200 toxins without any side effects. Licorice root is very sweet and is a great addition to herbal teas.

It helps regulate blood sugar levels and assists in neutralizing the effects of hypoglycemia; licorice also helps soothe any irritation in mucus membranes.

Finally, it relaxes muscles and is a natural muscle builder and strengthener.

Marshmallow Root

Marshmallow is a mild laxative as well as a diuretic. Its mucilaginous content provides relief for an irritated digestive tract as well as providing moisture to dry tissues.

Psyllium

An excellent source of dietary fiber. Psyllium is gluten free and is therefore a useful fiber source for those suffering from celiac disease or gluten intolerance.

It expands dramatically from the size of the original seeds and it is therefore essential to drink plenty of water with this product.

Psyllium absorbs toxins from the intestinal tract and binds them to fecal matter for elimination.

As it is a bulking agent, it often gives a feeling of fullness and discourages a person from over eating.

Violet Leaf

Is a good source of vitamin C and beta carotene (which the body converts to vitamin A as needed). Violet leaf has antifungal properties in addition to being a diuretic and laxative.

Yucca Root

Yucca root is high in fiber content and as such, is an excellent herb for digestive and intestinal problems. It can rid the body of undigested waste toxins which reside in the colon and cause foul smelling gases.

Historically, yucca root has been used as an anti-inflammatory and laxative agent that purges toxins from joints, which if left untreated, can cause inflammation that then leads to joint problems such as arthritis. Yucca is also effective at eliminating toxins from the blood, kidneys, liver and lymph.

Liver Support Herbs
Cascara Sagrada

Well known for it quick acting laxative effects. It is often used for constipation in addition to helping purge toxins from the body. It promotes peristaltic action—the movement of waste matter through the colon, and stimulates secretions from the gall bladder, liver, pancreas and stomach.

Dandelion

Dandelion has been used for centuries to stimulate the liver to detoxify poisons. It is important for promoting good circulatory system function and strengthening weak arteries.

Milk Thistle

One of the compounds in milk thistle—silymarin promotes the elimination of toxins from the liver. Milk thistle also protects the liver from the effects of substance abuse and alcohol consumption. It has anti-inflammatory properties to protect the liver from stress and injury.

Parasite Expulsion Herbs
Black Walnut

Black walnut is an excellent anti-parasitic herb, especially against worms. It also has high iodine content, which is good for energy as it supports thyroid function.

Garlic

Garlic is excellent for purging candida yeast and parasites from the body. Garlic has so many uses from using it in cooking to it being an excellent product for heart health. It also has antibacterial, anti-fungus and antiviral properties. Other recognized health benefits of garlic include, acting as an antibiotic and having anti-cholesterol and anti-hypertensive properties.

It is also an antioxidant which protects the body against the effects of free radical damage. Its high sulfur content assists in cell purification.

Allicin is the principle biological active compound which gives garlic its odor. Be warned. Many so called "odorless" garlic products have the active compound removed which makes it rather worthless. It can be obtained as a garlic bulb, in a capsule or in tablet form.

Pumpkin Seeds

One of the best tasting of all the anti-parasite herbal products. The seeds can be eaten as a snack. In fact they taste so good that you cannot eat enough of them. Pumpkin seeds are very effective against tapeworms as well as other types of parasites. They also serve as a good source of linolenic acid—one of the essential fatty acids (EFAs) which are essential for good health.

Herbs to Soothe an Irritated Digestive System and Urinary Tract
Cranberry

Cranberry's main purpose is to treat bacterial infections in the bladder. It is often combined with buchu herb.

Irish Moss

Irish moss is a type of seaweed that soothes an irritated gastro-intestinal tract. It is also used in hand and body lotion products to alleviate various skin conditions.

Passionflower

A natural sedative, passionflower will help you sleep without leaving a groggy feeling the next morning. It is beneficial for calming the nervous system and stress conditions.

Passionflower slows the breakdown of neurotransmitters which pass chemical messages between the body's cells, as well as working with certain enzymes. It also assists in calming an irritable bowel, as well as killing certain bacteria.

Herbs that have Antioxidant, Antiseptic and Anti-Inflammatory Properties
Capsicum

Also called cayenne pepper, this is the body's disinfectant. It helps rebuild tissue in the stomach as well as assisting in healing stomach and intestinal ulcers.

Capsicum has antioxidant and antiseptic properties in addition to providing support to the circulatory system. Its catalytic action helps in the transmission of other herbs to parts of the body where they are needed.

Chickweed

Chickweed is used to strengthen the colon and stomach as well as helping to dissolve plaque and fatty deposits. Chickweed has healing properties for stomach ulcers and inflammation in the colon.

Cranberry

Cranberry's main purpose is to treat bacterial infections in the bladder. It is often combined with buchu herb.

Gentian Root

Gentian root helps in the breakdown of fats and proteins and assists in the body's assimilation of iron and vitamin B12. As it has a cooling effect on body tissue, this helps reduce infections and inflammation. Gentian root also promotes digestive secretions.

Witch Hazel

Witch hazel has excellent anti-inflammatory and antiseptic properties. It has a high flavonoid content which helps to heal damaged blood vessels.

Herbs that Act as Blood Purifiers, Diuretics and Energy Providers
Burdock Root

Burdock root is one of the best blood purifiers to clear circulatory and lymphatic congestion. As it assists in alleviating excess body fluids, toxins are more easily purged from the body.

Other uses for burdock root: aids in reducing swelling around joints, expels surplus calcium deposits and cleanses the blood of harmful acids.

Chlorella

Chlorella contains over 19 amino acids. Of these, nine are the essential ones in addition to beta carotene (which the body converts to vitamin A as needed), potassium and other important vitamins and minerals, plus enzymes.

Chlorella has natural antioxidant properties and as such, is a good detoxifier, cell enhancer and blood cleanser.

When taken as a liquid it eliminates body odors from the digestive tract, and is also an excellent mouth wash to eliminate bad breath.

Echinacea

There are various strains of echinacea. It is used to support the immune system and is involved in the production of white blood cells, which assists the body in fighting infection. Echinacea purges toxins from the blood and enhances lymphatic drainage.

Fennel Seed

Fennel seed has several uses including: supporting the digestive and nervous systems, alleviating the effects of colic, gas and intestinal problems. It also has diuretic properties.

Fenugreek

Fenugreek is a respiratory system herb which assists in expelling mucous, phlegm and infections from the lungs, as well as toxic waste through the lymphatic system. In addition, fenugreek is able to dissolve a hardened build-up of mucous which can then be eliminated.

Garlic

Garlic is excellent for purging candida yeast and parasites from the body. Garlic has so many uses from using it in cooking to it being an excellent product for heart health. It also has antibacterial, anti-fungus and antiviral properties. Other recognized health benefits of garlic include, acting as an antibiotic and having anti-cholesterol and anti-hypertensive properties.

It is also an antioxidant which protects the body against the effects of free radical damage. Its high sulfur content assists in cell purification.

Allicin is the principle biological active compound which gives garlic its odor. Be warned. Many so called "odorless" garlic products have the active compound removed which makes it rather worthless. It can be obtained as a garlic bulb, in a capsule or in tablet form.

Ginger Root

Ginger root is an excellent cleansing agent for the colon, skin and kidneys. It provides support to the respiratory system. It is often used to alleviate the effects of a cold or flu. Many people take it as a "natural" product for motion and morning sickness.

Horsetail

Horsetail is one of the best herbs for improving digestion as well as relieving symptoms of bloating and gas.

As it is rich in trace minerals, it is an excellent herb for assisting the healing of the skin, bones and cartilage. As it is also an antifungal agent and diuretic it is a good herb in a detoxing program.

Mullein

A mucilaginous product which soothes irritated tissue. It is very beneficial for respiratory system health.

Oatstraw

Oatstraw is a good source of minerals for nourishing bones, hair, skin and nails.

It helps calm the nervous system and can assist in instances of depression and conditions of exhaustion.

Slippery Elm

Slippery elm is very soothing to inflamed tissue—especially in the gastrointestinal tract—and as a result, is excellent for tissue healing. It is easily digested and has good laxative properties.

Skin Cleansing Herbs
Burdock Root

Burdock root is one of the best blood purifiers to clear circulatory and lymphatic congestion. As it assists in alleviating excess body fluids, toxins are more easily purged from the body.

Other uses for burdock root: aids in reducing swelling around joints, expels surplus calcium deposits and cleanses the blood of harmful acids.

Capsicum

Also called cayenne pepper is the body's disinfectant. It helps rebuild tissue in the stomach as well as assisting in healing stomach and intestinal ulcers.

Capsicum has antioxidant and antiseptic properties in addition to providing support to the circulatory system. Its catalytic action helps in the transmission of other herbs to parts of the body where they are needed.

Colloidal Silver

This is available as a liquid or in gel form. Colloidal silver has been used for centuries to treat all manner of body conditions. It is especially useful for skin problems whether acquired through an injury or an infection. Colloidal silver gel makes a good general skin cleanser.

Ginger Root

Ginger root is an excellent cleansing agent for the colon, skin and kidneys. It also provides support to the respiratory system. It is often used to alleviate the effects of a cold or flu. Many people take it as a "natural" product for motion and morning sickness.

Oregano

Available in either enteric coated (meaning it will burst in the body where it is supposed to), or in liquid form, oregano possesses anti-inflammatory antiviral and anti-fungal properties and is an excellent herb for protecting the skin.

Peppermint Oil

Can be purchased as an enteric coated capsule or in liquid form. If liquid is used then only very tiny drops should be applied to water, otherwise it will be too strong. It is excellent for an upset stomach, to eliminate bad breath and as a general tonic.

Yellow Dock

Assists with elimination and is one of the best blood builders in the herbal arsenal.

I said this was a long list—I hope you have found it useful.

7. Start a 3-day detox diet

The 3-day detox diet is mainly used to purge your body of built up toxins that reside in your body systems. Toxins easily build up in the body through the effects of diet, as well as environmental factors. When toxins build up in your body it affects its ability to function properly, the effects of which often manifest themselves as feelings of sluggishness and lethargy.

This diet is accomplished by using natural fruits and vegetables that are uncooked. When you first start this diet you may be aware of some of the symptoms of the toxins as they leave your body. Some of these symptoms could include diarrhea and headache, or you could experience typical flu-like reactions. It is important to drink plenty of good quality filtered or bottled still water whilst you are on your detoxification program.

In addition, you should eliminate any caffeine products which include coffee, tea, and any soft drinks that contain caffeine. You should avoid eating anything that is cooked and stick only to fruits and vegetable sources. As an alternative, you may squeeze your juice and drink it if you prefer. It is also important that no artificial ingredients are consumed during your 3-day detox diet.

Try and avoid giving your body a routine. For instance, do not eat breakfast lunch and dinner at your normal times. Instead, let your body tell you when it is hungry and then only feed it with one type of fruit or vegetable at this time. Only eat until your body tells you that it has had enough. Do not eat until you are full.

When you get fed up with this one type of food item, then, choose a different one and so on. Eating a particular food item and deciding that you don't really want it anymore is your body's way of telling you, "I have had enough of this particular food", it will often feel less appealing than it was before, and for some reason it may also start to taste differently. In addition, other food items such as nuts may also be added for variety.

During your 3-day detox diet in addition to drinking adequate amounts of filtered water, it is also a good idea to add a multivitamin supplement into your diet if you're not already taking one, to help prevent any nutrient shortfall. It is also important to get adequate amounts of rest and sleep during this time.

As its name suggests, this detox diet should only be carried out for a period of 3-days. At the end of this period start to gradually add new foods back into your diet. If you add all the different foods back into your body at once, it could give it quite a shock. After your 3-day detox program your body should feel rejuvenated and your energy levels should have increased.

8. Detoxing The Juice Fast Way

So what is detoxing the juice fast way? Well, it involves eating raw fruit and vegetable juice and water for a specific period of time. As this is a rather intensive detoxing process, there are certain individuals who should avoid a juice fast detoxification program. These include pregnant or nursing mothers who put themselves and their baby at risk if they follow this program.

In addition, children should also avoid this type of detox program because their bodies are still growing, and they need an adequate amount of calories to enhance their growth process. Also, anyone should avoid a juice fast detox program prior to or immediately after surgery.

Other individuals who should avoid a juice fast detox program include those who have certain medical conditions including diabetes, kidney disease, liver disease or any other illness which affects the metabolic processes of the body. If however you are determined to pursue a juice fasting detox program with any of the above medical conditions, then it is imperative that you discuss this with your doctor first.

So what is involved in a juice fast detox program? Well, basically it consists of sipping between 32 and 64 ounces of juice spread throughout the day. These juices—which are best derived from organic sources—could include: carrot juice, apple juice, pineapple juice, cranberry juice, as well as cabbage, spinach, beets and greens. It is best if several fruits or vegetables are combined together to make a juice drink.

Citrus juices are usually avoided during a juice fast. And in addition to juices, it is also recommended that you drink at least six glasses of warm or room temperature filtered water each day as well.

Notice I do not mention tap water. Water companies in their infinite wisdom; tend to pollute drinking water which comes out of your tap with all manner of chemicals which the body then has to process. This extra processing causes additional stress on the body. And also, the body has to deal with all these extra chemicals before it can gain any benefit from the nutrients from the food you eat.

Typically a juice fast program will last between one to three days. If a longer timeline is proposed then a medical practitioner should be consulted to make sure that there are no nutritional deficits.

Once the juice fasting program has been concluded, it is important to reintroduce solid foods gradually; because if solid foods are introduced all at once, it could give the body systems quite a shock, which could have a negative effect on overall health.

Several side effects may be experienced which could include mild nutritional deficits or side effects from the detoxification process itself. Some common side effects could include acne, bad breath, body odor, constipation headaches and hypoglycemia.

Additional side effects may include diarrhea, dizziness, fainting, low blood pressure and vomiting. If you experience any of the side effects mentioned above while you are on a juice fast detox program, you should immediately stop the program and consult your doctor.

So what are the benefits of doing a juice fast detox program? Well, you could experience rapid weight loss. You could also notice a clearer skin, increased energy levels and an improvement in your digestive system.

One of the main advantages of doing a juice fast program is that you will eliminate toxins that have built up over time in your body systems, and it will also help your entire body function more efficiently. Various research is currently underway to determine how well the body responds to this type of fasting program and what types of health benefits you might get from such a program.

9. The Master Cleanse Diet—A Lemon Cleanse

The lemon cleanse is often called the Master Cleanse Diet and was first developed in 1941 by a healer who was self-taught named Stanley Burroughs. He made the claim that the lemon cleanse could be the one thing that would heal many different types of illnesses and diseases.

The Master Cleanse Diet (or lemon cleanse) was designed to aid in the removal of harmful toxins and poisons from the body

The Master Cleanse Diet consists of an all liquid diet which involves consuming 6 to 8 glasses of a drink which contains lemon juice, water, cayenne pepper and maple syrup. Here is a recipe for this drink:

For a single serving

2 Tablespoons of organic lemon Juice (approximately 1/2 a lemon)

2 Tablespoons of Organic grade B maple syrup (Do not use the commercial variety that is often used on pancakes)

1/10 Teaspoon Cayenne pepper powder

Ten ounces of filtered water

Mix all the ingredients together and consume

For a 60oz. daily serving:

12 Tablespoons of organic lemon juice

12 Tablespoons of organic grade B maple syrup

1/2 Teaspoon cayenne pepper powder

60 ounces of filtered water

Mix all the ingredients together and consume as required.

Note! It is important to use freshly squeezed lemon juice. Do not use the commercial variety from a tin or bottle. Also note the quality of the maple syrup is important too.

Stanley Burroughs asserted that maple syrup should be used because as it is rich in various vitamins and minerals. And lemons are defined as one of the most efficient cleansing and healing foods in alternative medicine.

The recommended time duration of the Master Cleanse Diet is 10 days. The individual isn't allowed to eat any other foods or liquids except water and the juice. It is literally a juice fast diet program.

And, to stimulate a daily bowel movement, the diet suggests participants should use an herbal laxative twice daily—morning and evening. Whilst on the diet participants shouldn't drink alcohol, cola, tea or coffee or smoke.

For the average person a day or two of fasting shouldn't have any ill effects. However, the Master Cleanse Diet involves at least 10 days of fasting and a calorie consumption of approximately 650 calories per day. Therefore, the dietary intake is especially low in protein, essential fats, vitamins and minerals—all of which are required for essential processes to maintain optimum body health. In addition, using laxatives to purge the body of toxins is also indicative of eating disorders.

By cycling the body between loss and gain, the heart, liver and kidneys can be placed under undue stress.

Once you're finished with the Master Cleanse Diet a specific procedure must be followed to break the fast. During the first day after completing this diet only orange juice should be consumed. During the second day you consume only orange juice again, but you can now include vegetable soup. On the third day after completing the cleanse you can have fruits, salads and vegetables. A normal diet can be resumed after day four.

People who have been on a Master Cleanse Diet have conflicting stories to tell. On the positive side, people who have used this diet state that they have more energy and a higher level of mental capacity. They also assert that they have an enhanced positive spiritual and psychological experience, which has the ability to improve their overall health

On the negative side, people who have been on the diet state that they experienced dizziness, felt faint and experienced severe hunger pangs. They also state that they had frequent bouts of diarrhea.

A word of caution! Anyone with serious health conditions such as cancer, diabetes or any type of intestinal structure as well as anyone with eating disorders should not follow this Master Cleanse Diet.

10. How About A Kidney Cleanse

A kidney cleanse simply means a detoxification of the kidneys. Kidney stones can be extremely painful, and if you have ever had them, then you will not want to repeat the experience. The purpose of a kidney cleanse is to dissolve any stones and flush out the tissues of the kidneys.

Some kidney stones can be more difficult than others to remove. Some can take several hours, while others can say several days or even months to get them to dissolve. So how are kidney stones formed? They are formed by crystals that accumulate inside the kidneys. These crystals consist of salts such as uric acid, cystines, xanthines as well as calcium oxalates.

The main cause of kidney stones is dehydration which arises through not drinking enough liquids, the result of which is that these salts become more concentrated. If these concentrations reach the point where they are not able to dissolve on their own, then, kidney stones will form.

Watermelons are excellent for use in a kidney cleanse. Eating several watermelons throughout the day will help to make you urinate more easily, as watermelon comprises mostly water. Alternatively, large amounts of liquid—and especially filtered water will be just as effective.

A juice fast which is explained in its own chapter can also be effective. If you use this method as a kidney cleanse then vegetable juice will be best in this case. You may also want to consider using herbs as part of a kidney cleanse. Herbs such as Ginger, Marshmallow Root, Parsley, Hydrangea, Goldenrod, Corn Silk Tea and Gravel Root have all proved to be effective as part of a kidney cleanse.

Increasing your intake of fluids and especially filtered water will be one of the best things you can do to help prevent kidney stones forming.

If you take Magnesium and Vitamin B6 supplements on a daily basis this could prove beneficial too. If your body has insufficient fluid intake then it finds it hard work to adequately digest any food you have consumed. And without adequate fluid intake you'll be more susceptible to develop constipation, cramping, gas as well as a feeling of being bloated.

There are several symptoms which can signal whether you have a kidney stone forming, these include pain—especially in the low back area, swelling and blood tinged urine. Low back pain in particular can be extremely excruciating, and something you will not want to repeat.

Having a prevention program in place is one of the best ways to guard against the formation of kidney stones. And if you are susceptible to them, than a twice yearly cleanse will be an appropriate action to take.

Some preventive things you should do include: avoid consumption of caffeine and any products that contain caffeine, reduce consumption of red meat and increase your fiber intake. Also reduce your salt consumption and avoid nuts, chocolate and dark green vegetables wherever possible.

11. How About Detox Foot Pads

Detox foot pads are the latest innovation in alternative health treatments. They are very simple to use. All you have to do is apply the pads to the soles of your feet at bedtime and the natural ingredients contained in these pads will draw out the toxins in your body through the soles of your feet while you sleep. Many people have tried these pads and have experienced relief from various joint pains as well as experiencing more relaxing sleep.

Ingredients in these foot pads will vary between different manufacturers, but in all cases the ingredients should be from natural sources which are not harmful to the body.

Wood vinegar is a natural ingredient that is often added to detox foot pads. Wood Vinegar has tremendous absorbing powers which helps relieve pain and decrease swelling in the body.

Bamboo vinegar is a tree sap that is extracted from bamboo and other broadleaf trees. It is processed using a rapid cooling technique which liquefies the sap, after which it is made into a vinegar solution. Bamboo vinegar will often be included in detox foot pads due to its ability to expel unwanted waste matter from the body.

Mugwort extract has been used for centuries to treat nervous conditions, as well as being a cure for insomnia and as an excellent liver stimulant. It has also been used successfully to treat various digestive disorders. As a result of all this, it is often included in detox foot pads.

The mineral Tourmaline is mined all over the world and is known as the "electric stone" because of the electric charge it naturally possesses. This electrical charge enables Tourmaline to produce far infrared photon energy, negative ions, and alpha waves. It is included as it has a cleansing effect on the body's nervous system.

The herb Loquat is often referred to as the king of herbal medicines. And it is often included in detox foot pads. The leaves of this herb contain various vitamins and acids. This herb's main benefits include enhancing secretions of body fluids as well as possessing anti-emetic and anti-tussive properties.

Eucalyptus oil is often included in the foot pads because of its very strong antibacterial and antiseptic properties. The leaves of the plant are used to reduce inflammation and fever.

Mixed results have been experienced by people have tried detox foot pads. Some individuals say they have had great success in using these pads to detoxify their body, and as a result they feel much better. Others say that detox foot pads are a con and they have gained no benefit from them whatsoever.

Current research suggests that whilst these foot pads might make you feel better, it has nothing to do with detoxifying your body, but is more to do with the effects of acupressure which is dependent on how you place the pads on the soles of your feet.

12. Parasite Infestations

A couple of years ago, I wrote a book titled *"An Easy Way To Understand Parasites, Worms, Candida, Constipation And Detoxing."* And this book has sold really well. All of which suggests that subjects covered in the book are of global concern.

In recent years researchers have spent much time evaluating the role that a healthy intestinal tract and colon plays in the general health of adults and children. Did you know that there are more than 100 different intestinal parasites that have been identified? So how do we describe a parasite? It is basically an organism that lives on or in another living organism and partially or wholly gets its nutrients from the host organism. This then can cause serious harm to the host while allowing the parasite to grow and multiply.

Parasite is a good name for these organisms, because what they basically are is a freeloader that resides in your body and take up the nutrients from your food which in reality should be going to nourish your body cells. These parasites release toxins which damage your body systems. Many researchers believe that over 40% of the world's population have a serious worm infestation. Worms are one of the commonest parasites that infest the colon.

So Where Do They Come From?

One of the questions that are often asked is "how can I possibly have a parasitic infection in my body and I am not aware of it"? This is how the parasite is so clever. It likes to keep a low profile because it knows if it is detected, then you'll make every effort to eradicate it.

We mistakenly think of parasitic infections as something that only happens in third world countries, but that is not the case. People in highly developed Western countries are just as at risk as less developed countries.

Given the fact that we are basically a global village these days with millions of people constantly flying across continents, in many ways it is not really surprising. Over the past few decades we have seen tens of thousands of people uproot themselves and move to the US and Europe especially. Often they bring parasites with them—as do soldiers returning from conflict zones overseas.

In many developed countries—despite all the precautions—many young children pick up parasites from day care centers. Even our pets also pose a big threat. Huge numbers of people pick up parasites from their cats and dogs. Going out to restaurants for meals can leave you more vulnerable than those who eat at home. Why? Because restaurant staff handling food are known to spread parasites—not deliberately, of course.

Some people are more likely to pick up parasites than others. People living in warm, humid areas have a greater risk. So do people in such jobs as animal handlers, plumbers, electricians, gardeners and sanitation workers as well as those who regularly travel abroad.

We can pick up parasites from all sorts of different places:

- Insect bites
- Animal feces
- Walking barefoot
- Handling raw meat and fish
- Eating raw or undercooked pork, beef or fish
- Handling soiled litter pans (cats)
- Eating contaminated raw fruits and vegetables
- Eating meals prepared by infected food handlers
- Drinking contaminated water
- Having contact with infected persons (including sexual contact, kissing and shaking hands)
- Inhaling contaminated dust (parasitic eggs or cysts)

13. Types of Parasites

First we need to understand exactly what they are, how they enter our body and what they do. Some parasites are tiny amoeba and protozoa which are so small you can only see them through a microscope. Others such as worms and flukes are much larger. But whatever their size, they still cause problems.

We normally only get infected by worms when we eat infected meat, fish or from our pets.

It's the amoeba and protozoa which pose the greatest degree of risk to us. They reach us through the air, via water, food, animals, insects and even human contact. They travel from our intestines and into our bloodstream, vital organs and muscles. Once lodged in these places they are free to cause maximum damage and often this can be considerable. They can be extremely infectious.

They've been linked to cancer, rheumatoid arthritis, asthma, diabetes, multiple sclerosis, pyorrhoea (a deterioration of the gums and the tissues surrounding your teeth) and other diseases.

Let's have a look at the main types of parasites, beginning with the ones we can normally see.

Worms

Pinworms

This is one of the most common types of worm. Although this worm sets up home in your colon, it lays its eggs outside your body. It means that you can pick up pinworms through unclean hands or dirty clothes and bed linen. You'll know if you've got it by the irritation and itchiness in your anal area.

Hookworms

This one lives in your intestines where it firmly attaches itself and proceeds to start sucking your blood. But it actually starts life outside your body in soil or water and this is how you get infected. Sometimes we pick it up by drinking water contaminated with hookworm larvae. Or it may get into our bodies via fruit or vegetables. The symptoms of having hookworms are general weakness, nausea, abdominal pain, diarrhea and anemia.

Roundworms

These are one of the most common parasites in the world and can be as large as a pencil. We absorb them into our system by ingesting eggs found in soil, fruit and vegetables. They start off in the intestine but then move off to attack other organs where they can do severe damage. If you've suffered weight loss, feel weak, have infections or find yourself with abdominal pain you may be infected.

Tapeworms

These are more common in cats and dogs than in people. To get infected you'd have to swallow the fleas which are themselves infected with tapeworm larvae. Like its cousins it takes up residence in the intestines where it steals vital nutrients and then excretes toxic waste into your gut. The big snag we face here is that people with tapeworms often don't show any symptoms. When they do it shows up as mineral deficiency problems, feeling bloated, dizziness, hunger pains, digestive problems, sensitivity to touch, allergies and not being able to think straight. A tapeworm can live inside the body for 25 - 30 years, and can grow to over 20 feet in length.

Liver fluke

These are particularly unpleasant. They attack your liver by drilling holes into it and causing inflammation. And—wait for it—these flukes can survive in your body for up to 30 years! You get them by eating undercooked fish, contaminated vegetables or human feces when it is used as fertilizer. It can also be acquired by drinking or swimming in contaminated water. It causes an enlarged liver, pains on the right side of the body, depression, edema (a build-up of fluid beneath the skin), vertigo, bile stones and in some cases cancer.

Protozoa

These come in a great many shapes and sizes but I will focus on the four most common types.

Giardia lamblia

Apart from pinworm this is about the most common type of parasite that affects humans. It is very widespread. These microbes hide in your intestine or gall bladder. It is spread through fecal contamination as well as through dirty water or unsafe sexual practices. It is resistant to chlorine, which means that you can still pick it up through tap water or from rivers and streams. Pains in your abdomen, sensitivity to food, diarrhea and vitamin deficiency are all symptoms.

Entamoeba histolytica

This is very tiny—just a single cell—but it causes a disease called amebiasis, an infection of the liver, intestines and other tissues. It is found in water and in damp places as well as in soil, vegetables and fruit. Again it can spread through fecal contamination, poor sanitation and unsafe sex as well as through crops fertilized with human waste. This parasite is especially difficult to detect as there aren't always symptoms, although in some warmer places it is the biggest killer after malaria. When symptoms do show up they appear as diarrhea, feelings of weakness, weight loss and pains in the abdomen.

Cryptosporidium

This one is often mentioned in the media especially when a hospital suffers an outbreak. It is another one-celled parasite which infects your digestive system and causes major gastro-intestinal upsets. Like the others, this one is spread through feces via the mouth. It is widespread throughout the environment and it can infect public water supplies as well as rivers and lakes. It can also be spread through restaurants, day care centers and unsafe sex. Diarrhea, flu-like symptoms and pains in your stomach are the tell-tale signs of an infection.

Toxoplasma gondii

This is a crescent-shaped invader which attacks your central nervous system. It gets into your body by eating under-cooked meat or handling infected cat litter which can contain its eggs. The truth is that most of us have been exposed to this parasite at some time so we have built up defences in the form of antibodies to counteract it. Therefore, only a few people actually show up with symptoms which tend to be flu-like, or you may experience fever, chills, tiredness and a headache.

14. Diagnosis And Symptoms

Although I have talked a little bit about the symptoms already, these infections are often very difficult to diagnose because the symptoms are extremely vague—or in some cases there are absolutely no symptoms at all.

If you feel unwell, here are some indications that you may have an infestation:

- Diarrhea with foul-smelling stool that becomes worse in the later part of the day
- Sudden changes in bowel habits (e.g. constipation that is now a soft and watery stool)
- Constant rumbling and gurgling in the stomach area unrelated to hunger or eating
- Heartburn or chest pain
- Flu-like symptoms such as coughing, fever, and nasal congestion
- Food allergy
- Itching around the nose, ears, and anus, especially at night
- Loss of weight with constant hunger
- Anemia
- Anxiety caused by the metabolic waste products of the parasites

But even this is not the end of the list because other symptoms could well include blood in the stool, bloating, diarrhea, gas, loss of appetite, intestinal obstruction and nausea. Other symptoms could include: vomiting, sore mouth and gums, excessive nose picking, grinding teeth at night, chronic fatigue, headaches, muscle aches and pains, shortness of breath, skin rashes, depression and memory loss.

Normally these kinds of infections are diagnosed by simply looking at stool samples under a microscope. Usually one of the public health laboratories undertakes this work.

The big problem is that traditionally there has been a high failure rate in identifying just what is wrong. So sometimes back up blood tests are needed as well. But when you think there are dozens of different types of parasites, you will understand that it is a big job identifying the correct ones.

Can There Be Complications?

Yes there can! But it is normally a problem that develops slowly. What happens is that worm populations build up over quite a long period of time. Eventually the health problems they cause get out of hand and become chronic.

For example, if you have got worms, you might suffer from malnutrition because they steal nutrients from your body and deprive you of the benefits of the nutrients from your food. Or it may be that they simply reduce your appetite. Either way, you are not getting what you need to stay healthy. If you have parasites in your system over a long period of time, it is likely to lead to food allergies.

Children who have got worms tend to be underweight and generally small for their age because worms have hampered their growth.

Roundworms can cause blockages in your colon. Intestinal worms, particularly hookworms can contribute to your having anemia because they cause loss of blood through bleeding in your intestines. The more worms you have got, the more problems you are likely to have.

Chronic parasite infections can be disastrous. They can stunt both your mental and physical development in the long term.

In some of the most severe cases they can even cause death.

15. How Do I Stop Myself Getting Infected With Parasites

Like many other things in life, it's a question of common sense. Here is a quick list of some of the more obvious measures:

- Wash your hands before eating and after using the toilet.

- Wear gloves when you are gardening or working with soil or sand because these can be contaminated with eggs or cysts of parasites.

- Pregnant women should avoid handling cat litter.

- Don't allow children to be licked or kissed by pets that are not wormed regularly.

- Wear long-sleeved shirts, long pants, and boots especially when walking through tall grass or amongst trees. In addition, spray insect-repellent on clothing to prevent tick bites.

- Have a regular curry which is an effective antidote to parasites. You can follow this with a probiotic supplement which helps to cleanse your intestines.

- You could consider a regular colon cleanse.

- Always wash your hands, kitchen counters and utensils with hot soapy water after cutting or handling raw meat, chicken or fish.

- Don't use a microwave to cook meat, chicken or fish. Microwaves often don't heat foods completely.

- Always wear shoes or slippers (to prevent hookworm infection).

- Do not use water from septic tanks or other potentially contaminated sources for watering vegetables

- Contain all fecal matter (for example, by using a toilet or latrine, rather than "as nature intended" outside).

- Teach children proper hygiene i.e. washing hands after going to the toilet, playing outside and before preparing or eating food.

- If you have parasites, you can reduce the likelihood of passing them on to others by carefully washing your hands after having bowel movements and cleaning the genital area before having sex.

- Wear gloves when changing the cat box. Make sure pets are wormed periodically.

- Avoid swallowing river, stream or lake water when swimming in them. Better yet, avoid swimming in them altogether.

- Keep your body slightly acidic by including pumpkin seeds, calimyrna figs, garlic, apple cider vinegar, cranberry juice and pomegranates in your diet.

- Avoid eating water chestnuts and watercress.

Remember that you don't need to wander barefoot across a garbage dump to pick up parasites. They're everywhere. So beware.

If one member of your family is treated then all other members should be treated as well because there can easily be cross-infections or re-infections. Make sure everyone washes their hands frequently and that bed linen, clothes and even soft toys are kept clean.

16. Some Dietary Guidelines
To Prevent Parasites

Eat as natural a diet as possible by buying organic meat, poultry, fruit and vegetables. Also include whole grains nuts and seeds. Make sure you get adequate fiber. Fiber assists in eradicating worms as well as toxins and chemicals from the intestines; and a good nutrition regime supports the immune system which helps protect the body against parasitic infection.

Here are a few important things to consider:

- Parasites thrive on dairy foods, fats and sugar so use these sparingly.

- Avoid eating raw or under-cooked fish, pork or beef. Remember these foods are a breeding ground for fish tapeworm, pork tapeworm and beef tapeworm respectively.

- Supplement your diet with a high quality natural multi-vitamin and multi-mineral supplement to ensure you don't have a dietary shortfall in essential nutrients. If your diet is lacking, then the body will utilize what it needs from the supplement. If your body doesn't need it, then it will pass out in the urine.

- Make sure you have adequate "friendly" bacterial in your intestinal tract, especially if you have taken a course of antibiotics. Antibiotics not only kill harmful bacteria, but friendly bacteria too. A good probiotic supplement containing Lactobacillus Acidophilus and other beneficial bacteria will ensure normal intestinal flora function which will help stop parasites from spreading.

17. Drug Treatment And Cure For Parasites

The traditional way to treat parasites is by using a variety of drugs. This works on the basis of something we call "differential toxicity". All that means is that the drugs are more poisonous to the parasite than they are to you—hopefully. It doesn't always work out that way and there can be side-effects from these drugs such as nausea, abdominal pains, vomiting, headaches and rashes.

Depending on how severe your infection is, you'll probably be provided with one of the following medications:

Albendazole

Albendazole is an anti-worm medication, and is used to treat certain infections caused by worms especially pork tapeworm and dog tapeworm. It prevents newly hatched insect larvae (worms) from growing or multiplying in the body.

Furazolidone

Furazolidone is taken by mouth and works in the intestinal tract. The drug is used to treat such conditions as cholera, colitis, and/or diarrhea caused by bacteria, giardiasis and protozoa. Protozoa are tiny, one-celled creatures some of which are parasites that if left untreated are the cause of many different kinds of infections in the body.

Iodoquinol

This medication is used to treat certain parasite infections in the intestines. It is either used alone or combined with other medications. It is not recommended to use this medication to treat a diarrhea condition where the cause is not determined.

Mebendazole

This medication is used to prevent worms such as hookworm, pinworm, roundworm and whipworm from growing and multiplying in the body.

Metrodidazole

This is an antibiotic which is used to treat a protozoa parasite infection.

Niclosamide

Niclosamide is used to treat various tape worm infestations such as beef tapeworm, dwarf tapeworm and fish tapeworm. It works by killing tapeworms on contact. The dead worms are then passed out in the feces. This medication will not work on other types of worms such as pinworms and roundworms.

Paromomycin

Paromomycin is an antibiotic which is used to treat various intestinal infections, as well as certain liver problems.

Pyrantel pamoate

This medication works by paralysing the nervous system of certain worms such as pinworm and roundworm which are then passed out in the feces.

Pyrimethamine

Pyrimethamine is used to prevent the growth and reproduction of parasites.

Quinacrine

Quinacrine is used in the treatment of the protozoa giardiasis in the intestinal tract.

Sulfadiazine

Sulfadiazine is an antibiotic, which is used to fight bacterial infections in the body.

Thiabendazole

Thiabendazole is a treatment used to prevent worms—such as threadworm from growing and multiplying in the body. In addition it may also be used to treat pinworm where this occurs with hookworm, roundworm, threadworm and whipworm.

18. Herbal Products For Parasites
An Alternative Method

Luckily, there are also much more gentle ways of dealing with lingering parasites such as herbal remedies, normally taken on an empty stomach before meals. You'll find a wide variety in shops and on the Internet. I have included a list below.

Black Walnut

Black walnut is an excellent anti-parasitic herb, especially against worms. It also has an high iodine content, which is good for energy as it supports thyroid function.

Cloves

Cloves are a good natural parasite cleansing herb which can be obtained as a liquid, powder or in a capsule.

Colloidal Silver

Although not a herb, colloidal silver has many uses and has been found to be effective against many surface micro-organisms, viruses, protozoa, amoeba, fungi, parasites and yeasts.

There are many different colloidal silver products on the market. You need to source one that contains 99.9 percent pure silver without any additives other than purified water.

Grapefruit Seed Extract

Grapefruit seed extract is an effective anti-parasitic herb which has a very bitter taste. This can be sweetened by adding a small amount of honey.

Garlic

Garlic has so many uses from using it in cooking to it being an excellent product for heart health. It also has antibacterial, anti-fungus and antiviral properties. Other recognized health benefits of garlic, include acting as an antibiotic as well as other health advantages like its anti-cholesterol and anti-hypertensive properties.

It is also an antioxidant which protects the body against the effects of free radical damage. Its high sulfur content assists in cell purification.

Allicin is the principle biological active compound which gives garlic its odor. Be warned. Many so called "odorless" garlic products have the active compound removed which makes it rather worthless. It can be obtained as a garlic bulb, in a capsule or in tablet form.

Pumpkin Seeds

One of the best tasting of all the anti-parasite herbal products. The seeds can be eaten as a snack. In fact they taste so good that you cannot eat enough of them. Pumpkin seeds are very effective against tapeworms as well as other types of parasites. They also serve as a good source of essential fatty acids (EFAs) which are important for good health.

Essential Fatty Acids

Essential Fatty Acids are so called because you have to get them from your diet—the body cannot make them itself. There are two essential fatty acids: omega-3 and omega-6. These two are the building blocks that make the twenty fatty acids that the body needs for good health.

Essential fatty acids are important for the manufacture of cell membranes as well as important hormones and neurotransmitters—chemical substances that pass messages between different cells which tell the body what to do.

They are also involved in the manufacture of prostaglandins in your body. These hormone-like substances help control many different activities. Some of these activities include such things as inflammation, pain, and unbelievably, some cause swelling and some reduce swelling. They are involved in allergic reactions, blood clotting and the manufacture of other hormones.

Prostaglandins also have a role to play in controlling blood pressure, heart and kidney function, body temperature in addition to being involved in the digestive system.

Being natural blood thinners, fatty acids help prevent blood clots, which can trigger a heart attack and stroke.

Arthritis and autoimmune diseases can be relieved by the natural anti-inflammatory compounds found in essential fatty acids.

If you experience skin problems such as dull or brittle hair, if your nails split easily, or you have dandruff or eczema, then your diet could be lacking in essential fatty acids.

Essential Fatty Acids have an important role to play in good digestive and intestinal systems health. They help maintain cell stability in addition to increasing the thickness of cells lining the intestinal tract, as well as the villi which enhances the absorption of nutrients. All this leads to better digestion and improved health.

19. Let's Not Forget Constipation

Would you believe that's over 4 million Americans will suffer from frequent constipation this year. It is one of the most frequent gastro-intestinal complaints in the United States today. Statistics show that individuals aged 65 or older and women are the most likely candidates to suffer from constipation.

Women will often become constipated while pregnant, and it is not uncommon to become constipated following delivery of a baby. In older people, many become constipated due to medications that they are taking for various health issues, in addition to reduced fluid intake and lack of activity.

So how do you define constipation? Individuals will often define constipation as not having a bowel movement every day. However, medical professionals define constipation as not having a bowel movement for three or more consecutive days. In the normal range, the number of bowel movements is assessed as between twice a day and every other day. In fact, individuals who consume the recommended amount of fiber and drink enough fluids each day will in all probability have a bowel movement every day and possibly twice a day.

When an individual is constipated they will have difficulty having a bowel movement—and it can be very painful to expel stools because they will become small, hard and dry. As a result of being constipated, these individuals may feel bloated and have a sensation that their bowel is fully loaded.

Constipation is not a disease but is really a symptom which can be treated very easily in most cases. Most cases are caused by the following: a lack of fiber in the diet, a lack of physical activity, and not drinking enough fluids with the result that the body becomes dehydrated, and ignoring a bowel urge because the individual might be too busy to deal with it. Another cause of constipation can be the misuse of laxative products. Excess use of laxatives can damage the nerve endings in the colon making it virtually impossible to have a normal bowel movement.

Some diseases can cause constipation as well. These include neurological conditions, metabolic conditions and endocrine conditions.

These conditions can reduce the rate of movement of the stools from the colon, rectum and anus. This has the effect of making stools very hard and difficult to pass.

If you're constipated it is important to determine the cause before commencing any treatment. But in most cases various things can be done to ease the problem. For mild constipation, simple dietary changes can often eradicate the problem. If your diet contains 20 to 35 grams of dietary fiber per day this will help the body to form soft bulky stools which will be easier to eliminate. A qualified dietician should be consulted for information on which foods to eat which should increase the amount of fiber in the daily diet.

Increasing the intake of water as well as increasing activity levels can help alleviate constipation. Water in addition to fruit and vegetable juices will help to keep you hydrated which has the effect of reducing instances of constipation. It is also very important to make sure that you allow sufficient time to have a good bowel movement. When you ignore the urge to go because you are too busy, the stool will stay in the large intestines for an excessive amount of time with the result that more water will be removed and the stool with become hard, making it more difficult for it to be eliminated.

If dietary changes and an increased activity level do not seem to work, then your physician may suggest the use of laxatives for a short period of time. Laxatives should not be used for lengthy periods of time because they can increase your chances of becoming constipated with the result that problems can be caused with the intestines leaking bacteria and viruses into the bloodstream.

20. Notice To Readers

Some of the herbal products mentioned in this book may not be available in your country due to misguided government regulatory reasons, or an attempt by regulatory agencies to deny your choice of using "natural" products as opposed to drug based medications.

If this applies to your country, then you can always try the Internet. In this enlightened age of global communications, at the touch of a button, with a little effort on your part, you can often find the products that you require, and most suppliers will ship their products globally.

21. Resources

Good Colon Health

Michigan Bowel Control Program: Constipation
   http://www.med.umich.edu/bowelcontrol/patient/constipation.shtml

MedlinePlus: Colon Cancer
   http://www.nlm.nih.gov/medlineplus/ency/article/000262.htm

American Cancer Society: Colorectal Cancer Overview
   http://www.cancer.org/cancer/colonandrectumcancer/
overviewguide/colorectal-cancer-overview-what-causes

MayoClinic: Dietary Fiber
   http://www.mayoclinic.com/health/fiber/NU00033

Start A 3-Day Detox Diet GaiamLife: 3 Day Clean Food Detox Plan
   http://life.gaiam.com/article/3-day-clean-food-detox-plan

Consider A Cleansing Diet

Dr. Frank Lipman: Detox Demystified
   http://www.drfranklipman.com/
detox-demystified-fad-fact-or-fiction/

University of Wisconsin School of Medicine: Detoxification to Promote Health
   http://www.fammed.wisc.edu/sites/default/files//webfm-uploads/
documents/outreach/im/handout_detoxplan.pdf

Detoxing The Juice Fast Way

Boston.com: Taking a Break From Eating
   http://www.boston.com/lifestyle/health/articles/2012/03/12/
taking_a_break_from_eating/?page=1

Cornell University: Study on fasting and dieting suggests why diets fail -- and why a weekly fast might work
   http://news.cornell.edu/stories/2010/03/
study-fasting-suggests-why-diets-fail

University of Southern California: Fasting Makes Brain Tumors More Vulnerable to Radiation Therapy
   http://www.sciencedaily.com/releases/2012/09/120911172308.htm

Dr. Ben Kim: Is Fasting One Day a Week Good For Your Health
http://drbenkim.com/fasting-fast-one-day-week.htm

The Master Cleanse Diet—A Lemon Cleanse
Natural News: The Lemon Detox Diet
http://www.naturalnews.com/035854_lemons_detox_recipe.html

How About A Kidney Cleanse
National Kidney and Urologic Disease Information
Clearinghouse: Diet for Kidney Stone Prevention
http://kidney.niddk.nih.gov/kudiseases/pubs/kidneystonediet/in-dex.aspx

National Kidney and Urologic Disease Information
clearinghouse: Kidney Stones in Adults
http://kidney.niddk.nih.gov/kudiseases/pubs/stonesadults/

Mercola: Who Knew Preventing Kidney Stones was this Easy?
http://articles.mercola.com/sites/articles/archive/2009/06/23/Who-Knew-Preventing-Kidney-Stones-was-This-Easy.aspx

How About Detox Foot Pads
Mercola: Detox Foots Pads a Scam
http://articles.mercola.com/sites/articles/archive/2008/10/14/detoxifying-foot-pads-are-a-scam.aspx

Parasites In The Colon
(1) American Family Physician: Common Intestinal Parasites
http://www.aafp.org/afp/2004/0301/p1161.html

(2) University of Maryland Medical Center: Intestinal Parasites
http://www.umm.edu/altmed/articles/intestinal-parasites-000097.htm

Let's Not Forget Constipation
National Digestive Diseases Information Clearinghouse:
Constipation
http://digestive.niddk.nih.gov/ddiseases/pubs/constipation/

MayoClinic: Constipation
http://www.mayoclinic.com/health/constipation/DS00063/DSECTION=treatments-and-drugs

University of Michigan Health System: Constipation
http://www.med.umich.edu/bowelcontrol/patient/index.shtml?gclid=CPa1ncqrubMCFSXNOgodHDIAkQ

About The Author

Brian B Jacques started in business at a young age, and over the ensuing years, he has developed several very successful businesses. But his main interest for the past 40 years has been in natural health research and publishing.

Brian has presented seminars worldwide on such diverse subjects as Health Related issues, Motivation and Personal Development. In addition he has written numerous books, newsletters and articles on these subjects.

His very popular series of Mini Health Books has circulated widely around the world, and many more titles are in preparation.

Brian is a highly motivated individual, so much so that in 1985 he received a UK Industrial Society award for his work in the Motivation and Personal Development fields.

Brian has the following mottos:

- If something does not work out for you, then don't give up, but keep trying, trying, trying until finally you succeed.

- Success or failure in any endeavor is in your own hands.

Brian and his wife divide their time between East Yorkshire, UK and Florida, USA.

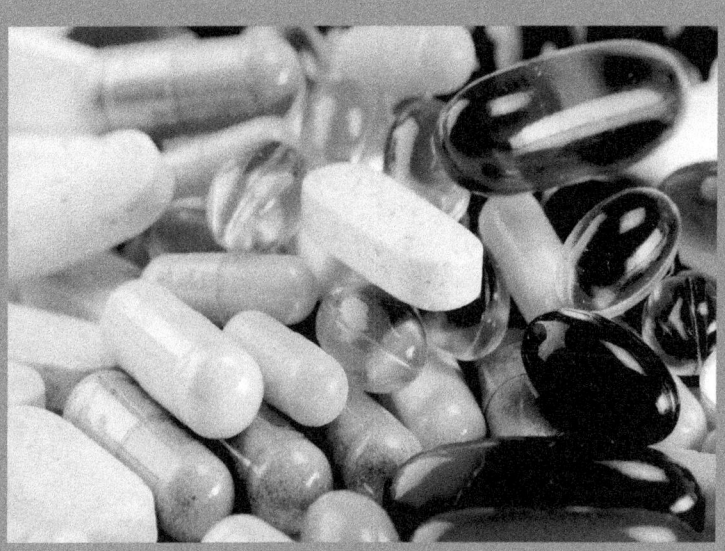

www.ingramcontent.com/pod-product-compliance
Lightning Source LLC
Chambersburg PA
CBHW071113280526
45787CB00003B/1014